CW00350440

The Powe
for Men

(Building Strength and Flexibility
Like Never Before)

Copyright@2023

Victor Pandevis

Chapter one
What is Pilates?

Pilates exercises encompass both bodyweight matwork and equipment-based workouts, demanding your utmost attention and dedication.

Matwork sessions involve deliberate movements while lying on your back or stomach, where you engage your core muscles intensely for functional support. Gravity serves as your unwavering adversary, pushing you to sustain spinal and joint mobility while fortifying the intricate muscles that maintain your body's alignment.

For an extra challenge, Pilate's aficionados turn to spring-based equipment like the reformer, stability chair, Cadillac or tower, and a set of barrels, amplifying the potential for transformation.

While ongoing research is essential, emerging studies strongly hint at the manifold benefits of Pilates: enhancing strength and flexibility, mitigating nonspecific low back pain, regulating glucose levels, alleviating arthritis discomfort, sharpening balance and gait, elevating athletic performance, and, remarkably, uplifting one's mood.

Over the years, men have traditionally emphasized specific muscle groups in their weightlifting endeavors, often obsessing over chest, biceps, and the coveted "six-pack" abs.

Enter Pilates, either as a supplement to your strength training routine or a standalone fitness regimen, to rectify the imbalances wrought by this overzealous focus. Pilates seamlessly integrates into a comprehensive fitness strategy, encompassing aerobic exercise, traditional strength training, and a balanced diet.

Pilates, notably, fosters profound core strength in men, diligently addressing muscular disparities and their accompanying discomforts. Embrace Pilates as a powerful tool for achieving equilibrium and cultivating a pain-free existence.

Chapter Two

A Brief History of Pilates: Empowering Men's Fitness

While contemporary fitness marketing predominantly spotlights Pilates as a women-centric pursuit, it's high time to acknowledge that men stand to gain extraordinary benefits from these exercises as well.

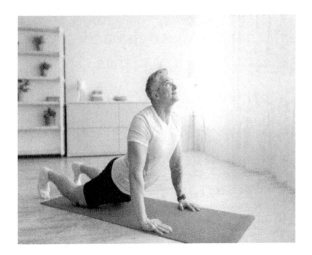

Let's rewind to the genesis of this transformative discipline: Pilates, not a woman, but a resolute German man by the name of Joseph Pilates, pioneered it in the early 20th century.

Joseph Pilates, in his youth, battled formidable health challenges, grappling with afflictions like asthma and rickets. He possessed an unyielding determination to fortify his physique, propelling him into a lifelong odyssey through an eclectic array of physical pursuits. He embraced martial arts, sculpted his body through bodybuilding, exhibited grace in gymnastics, and even stepped into the boxing ring.

During a fateful stint with a traveling circus amid the tumultuous backdrop of World War I, Pilates found himself interned as a foreign national on the Isle of Man. It was within this internment that the seeds of the Pilates method were sown. Pilates, leveraging his ingenuity, ingeniously rigged the earliest iteration of the Pilates Cadillac machine, ingeniously fashioning it from springs attached to hospital beds.

The impact was nothing short of miraculous. Soldiers, recuperating from their wartime injuries, who partook in Pilates' innovative training regimen recovered with astonishing speed, outpacing their counterparts who were not exposed to this transformative approach.

But Joseph Pilates' heroics didn't end there. Amid the ravages of the Spanish Flu pandemic, he shouldered the responsibility of maintaining the health of the 24,000 men confined within the camp. He orchestrated daily exercise routines and assumed the role of an orderly in the camp hospital. The legend that endures is one of resilience: not a single soldier under his care succumbed to the grip of the deadly flu.

The history of Pilates is undeniably a tale of unyielding determination, innovative genius, and transformative results, and it is a legacy that unequivocally extends its manifold benefits to men on a quest for fitness and well-being.

For what reason should men think about Pilates?

Maybe due to how Pilates is showcased or the famous impression of Pilates, individuals frequently partner this exercise technique with ladies.

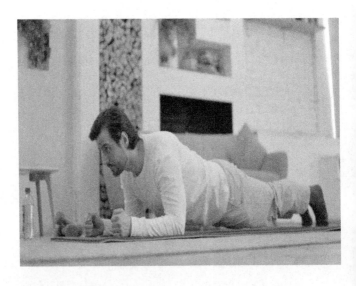

In any case, despite the fact that Pilates is promoted toward a particular orientation, its advantages are, generally, the equivalent for men concerning ladies.

The greatest contrast in advantages of Pilates for men as contrasted and ladies lies in the propensity for men to prepare in a manner that overemphasizes specific muscle bunches in their exercises and ignores other muscle gatherings.

It has been proven by Pilates teacher and prime supporter of Kinected and the Utilitarian Life structures for Development and Wounds studio, Pilates can assist men with figuring out how to track down balance in their exercises.

"Men tend to overtrain certain joints, locales, and muscles, for example, the rectus abdominis 'six-pack muscle,' the biceps and rear arm muscles, and the quads. Because of this overtraining and resultant solid unevenness, men will generally cause specific incessant wounds."

Research has it that men frequently stall out in the preparation schedules they learned in secondary school and spotlight just on incorporating greater muscles as opposed to on bringing the body into equilibrium and arrangement via preparing the characteristic muscles as well.

"Pilates is like a system that helps fix any issues in your body by making it stronger and more flexible, which also improves how efficiently it works," he explains. "When your body is well-balanced and your muscles work efficiently, you're less likely to get injured."

How common is the act of Pilates among men?

Pilates is encountering a developing prevalence among men, enveloping different socioeconomics including competitors, wellness lovers, and working experts who look to check the unfriendly impacts of delayed times of sitting.

As indicated by research, "At first, Pilates was dominatingly promoted towards ladies and related basically with artists. Be that as it may, this discernment has advanced altogether. Proficient competitors from different games, have integrated Pilates into their preparation schedules, breaking old generalizations and featuring the flexibility of Pilates, which has reverberated with an assorted scope of people, not simply men."

Strong Pilates Routine Custom-made for Men

Release Your Internal Strength with These Crucial Activities!

Get ready to handle your awkward nature head-on with this powerful Pilates routine extraordinarily made for men. Try not to misjudge its viability; this routine ought to be embraced with assurance 2-3 times each week, on days separated.

Chapter Three

The Hundred: Revive Your Center and Cardiovascular Framework

The Hundred is a quintessential Pilates mat activity, employing unmatched ability to light your body and supercharge your heart and circulatory framework.

For what reason is it ideal for men, you inquire? Now is the ideal time to expel those secondary school-period crunches that have caused more damage than great. As indicated by McCulloch, crunches have prompted neck snugness and overtraining of the six-pack muscles, eventually yielding restricted benefits.

To set out on The Hundred:

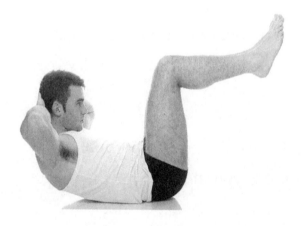

Start by leaning back on your back on an agreeable mat.

Raise your head and shoulders off the mat while drawing your knees toward your chest.

Push your legs to a high corner to corner position, with arms stretched out close by your body, palms confronting.

Overwhelmingly siphon your arms, guaranteeing they rise no higher than your hip's culmination.

All the while, breathe in profoundly for a determined 5-second range, trailed by a breathe out of equivalent span.

Rehash this 5-second breathe in and breathe out cycle a stunning multiple times, gathering a fabulous all out of 100 counts.

Change the activity's force by flexing or completely expanding your legs. Keep in mind, the vital lies in drawing in your muscular strength without stressing your neck or bending your back.

Embrace this extraordinary Pilates schedule, recover your equilibrium, and reveal your actual potential!

The Shoulder

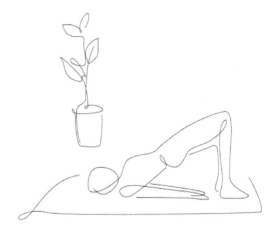

The Shoulder Extension is a flat
out force to be reckoned with in
the realm of Pilates, a unique
advantage that requests your
consideration. It's not just about
reinforcing; about rebalancing
your body in a way can't be

disregarded, especially for the fellas out there.

Let this hit home: Your quads and hip flexors, those frequently exhausted muscles that can torment men with knee-following issues, meet their match in the Shoulder Extension. Everything without question revolves around harmony. Get ready to observe the change as it braces your gluts, limbers up those obstinate hip flexors, and produces an unshakable center.

Presently, how about we separate it. To vanquish the Shoulder Extension:

Begin your back, legs bowed, feet hip-width separated. Keep your arms immovably at your sides, palms down.

As you breathe out, gather your internal solidarity to lift your pelvis and hips. The outcome? A dynamic, corner to corner line extending from knee to bear. For an additional portion of center ability, hoist yourself by flexing your spine, beginning from the tailbone and climbing to the ribs.

One leg, completely straight, ascents magnificently toward the sky while your pelvis stays level.

Let it all out! Raise and lower that leg in the air, threefold finished.

Tenderly curve the drawn out knee and return to your underlying position.

Presently, remember to equally spread the adoration. Rehash this brilliant activity on the two sides, exchanging with each wonderful reiteration.

Could five reps on each side? Trust us; it's the enchanted number.

Need to dial it down an indent? Don't worry about it. Just avoid the leg lift and lower or keep the two feet fixed solidly on the floor.

Plan to meet your match, Shoulder Scaffold style. It's not only an exercise; an extraordinary encounter places

your body fitting together.
Embrace the test!

The Swan

The Swan is an Outright
Fundamental in Pilates matwork,
a genuine huge advantage that
will Change your spine and
Rejuvenate your stance! This
exercise is the distinct advantage
against the feared adjusted back
droop that torment the
individuals who go through hours
sitting.

Tune in up, in light of the fact
that this is an Unquestionable

requirement for everybody, particularly you folks out there! Most men totally disregard spinal augmentation in their exercises, however in the event that you're holding back nothing MUSCLE Equilibrium, THIS is your ticket! The Swan will Raise your back strength and Release your spinal Portability, opening another degree of Actual Essentialness. Not any more falling into those T. rex-like stances we see wherever these days!

Presently, how about we get serious. To Dominate the Swan:

Begin by lying Level on your stomach, preparing to Release the power inside.

Twist those elbows and KEEP them near your sides. PALMS immovably established close to your shoulders, and LEGS hip-distance separated for that Unshakable BASE. In the event that you're feeling Courageous, go more extensive for some Additional Security!

PRESS into the ground like you would not joke about this! Draw in those UPPER-BACK muscles

and LIFT your HEAD,
SHOULDERS, and CHEST OFF THE
MAT. Keep those ABS TIGHT and
your SPINE Extended, no space
for loosen! Initiate those GLUTES
and HAMSTRINGS to keep those
FEET Immovably on the floor.

Lower down Leisurely, each
VERTABRA in turn, since we do
nothing apathetic!

What's more, here's the kicker -
do it not once, not two times, but
rather 5 REPS! That is the way
you come by RESULTS.

Feeling like you really want a few changes? Don't sweat it!

To make it a piece Simpler, spread those LEGS out and turn those KNEES and TOES to the sides. Along these lines, you get considerably MORE GLUTE Activity.

Need to Wrench UP the power? Unite those LEGS or have a go at keeping that Lengthy SHAPE as you LIFT your HANDS and ROCK FORWARD.

That's the main idea - The Swan offers a surefire solution for improving your posture. It's time to dive into the world of strong and flexible spines so you can excel in your physical activities and leave injuries behind. You might even start feeling as graceful as a swan among a group of ducks.

THE SIDE BEND: UNLEASH THE FULL POTENTIAL OF YOUR SPINE!

Prepare to experience spine liberation like never before with the Side Bend—an exercise that pushes your spinal flexibility to the extreme! This is no ordinary workout; it's a game-changer that takes your spine on a thrilling journey through lateral flexion, a realm seldom explored in conventional training. Your spine is a marvel, designed to bend in all directions, including sideways. Neglecting this crucial range of motion can spell trouble down the road, and you definitely don't want that.

According to the expert, the Side Bend unleashes the full potential of your spine by allowing it to gracefully glide through multiple planes. Forget the mundane, one-dimensional routines typical of traditional male workouts. This exercise is a revelation—it not only ramps up your shoulder mobility and stability but also supercharges your trunk rotation. And here's a golden nugget: it's a secret weapon for improving your golf game! Yes, you heard that right.

So, brace yourself for a spine-transforming experience with the Side Bend. It's time to awaken the dormant potential of your spine and revolutionize your fitness routine.

To conquer the Side Bend:

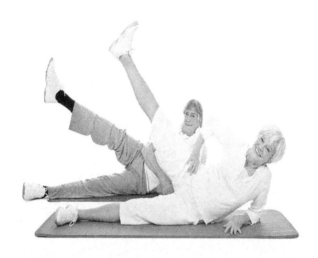

Take your position: Get seated on your trusty mat, and make a bold statement by shifting your weight onto one hip. For this demonstration, let's dive in with your left hip on the mat.

Left hand at the ready: Place your left hand flat on the floor next to you, asserting dominance with that straight arm.

Bend those knees: It's time to get those knees in on the action. Rotate your right knee towards the heavens and firmly plant your right foot flat on the mat. Keep your left leg bent, resting regally on the mat, with the shin proudly positioned in front of you and the knee open wide. Cross your right ankle over your left, ensuring that the right heel cozies up to the left ankle.

Prepare for the rise: Let your right arm relax by your side and take a deep, empowering breath in.

The ascent: With the force of a champion, exhale and push into your feet and that steadfast left hand simultaneously. Feel your bottom hip gracefully lift off the mat. Straighten those legs, guiding your left shoulder over the left hand, and let your body curve towards the heavens, creating a breathtaking arch or a vibrant rainbow within your spine.

Align with perfection: Keep your head, shoulders, ribs, pelvis, knees, and feet all in perfect harmony, dancing along the same electrifying lateral plane.

The return: Inhale triumphantly as you gracefully return to your starting position, ready for the next exhilarating round.

Repeat the magic: Don't stop there! Aim for 6–8 repetitions of this spine-awakening masterpiece. And when you're done, don't forget to switch sides

and embark on the journey all
over again.

Get ready to unlock the hidden
potential of your spine, and let
the Side Bend be your gateway to
a world of spine-tingling fitness!

Leg Pull Front

The Leg Pull Front is an intense
core strength exercise that
absolutely engages every area of
your body.

This dynamic Pilates move doesn't just stop at the plank position; it takes it to the next level by incorporating a precise foot, ankle, and leg raise, all while maintaining perfect balance on the opposing leg.

According to research, "Focusing on shoulder stability should be the top priority for most men before ramping up their reps in exercises like pushups, which are crucial for building shoulder and chest strength."

But here's the kicker – Leg Pull Front doesn't just work on shoulder stability; it's a complete powerhouse, enhancing your shoulder stability, core strength, hip strength, and yes, even your ankle strength and flexibility. Why is this important? Well, it's your ticket to acing those long runs when the mercury rises and, more importantly, shielding yourself from potential lower back, foot, and ankle issues.

Now, let's get down to business and master the Leg Pull Front:

Commence in a high plank position. Your abdominals should be as tight as a drum, and your feet should be glued together, with a significant portion of your weight resting on the balls of your feet. Keep those hips, shoulders, and ears in pristine alignment – they should be as straight as an arrow.

Inhale deeply, and with precision, extend one leg from the hip, raising your foot just a few inches off the mat. As that leg ascends, concentrate fiercely on keeping your hips rock-solid and preventing any unwanted shifts.

This isn't just an exercise; it's a symphony of core stabilization, shoulder engagement, and a back workout that means business.

Exhale forcefully while pointing your foot and ankle, simultaneously shifting your weight backward through space. Feel that supporting leg's ankle flex as you maintain that unwavering core and shoulder control.

Inhale with intent, shifting forward again on the supporting foot, all while flexing that lifted foot as if you're sculpting every muscle.

Now, exhale purposefully as you lower your foot back to the floor, returning to the original starting position. Your body should be a picture of power and precision throughout.

Don't settle for just one side; repeat relentlessly, alternating each repetition, ensuring that you complete a total of 10 reps on each side. It's not just about strength; it's about balance and endurance.

As you embark on this exercise journey, sternly reject any notion of your lower back sagging. And remember, your feet are your foundation; distribute your body weight evenly to maintain that unbreakable form.

If, for any reason, you find it impossible to maintain the spine's integrity while executing the full exercise, don't despair – simply hold that plank position, and you'll still be working wonders for your core.

Chapter Four
Life-Enhancing Benefits of Pilates

Pilates, the pinnacle of neuromuscular full-body functional training, boasts an array of meticulously researched advantages that elevate both physical prowess and mental well-being to remarkable heights.

Harnessing the profound "mind-body" connection it champions, consistent Pilates practice emerges as a potent enhancer of executive function, an accolade not to be underestimated (10).

For our cherished older generation, the practice of Pilates is nothing short of transformative, gifting them with newfound balance, coordination, and mobility, fortifying their defenses against the looming specter of falls that can accompany aging (11).

Intriguingly, research resoundingly heralds Pilates as a panacea for chronic nonspecific back pain, a pervasive ailment afflicting a staggering 80 percent of the populace (1Trusted Source).

Furthermore, Pilates training reigns supreme when pitted against yoga, showcasing marked improvements in functional movement screen (FMS) assessments. These include a battery of seven pivotal tests like the deep squat, lunges, hurdle steps, shoulder mobility, and straight leg raises—a testament to its efficacy in enhancing everyday functionality and athletic prowess (12Trusted Source).

A captivating revelation from a study involving young men unraveled Pilates' profound impact on psychological well-being. A mere 30-minute Pilates matwork session yielded tangible reductions in anxiety and fatigue, underscoring its potential as a psychological tonic (3).

And for those in pursuit of cardiovascular vigor, the evidence is resounding—Pilates training bestows heightened performance on submaximal aerobic tests, even among those who typically

steer clear of aerobic endeavors
(13).

Lastly, a groundbreaking 2020 study illuminated Pilates as a potent antidote to hypertension. Individuals grappling with elevated blood pressure experienced an acute drop in readings following a solitary Pilates session, offering a tantalizing glimpse into its potential as a formidable weapon against this pervasive health concern (14).

In the realm of fitness and well-being, Pilates stands as a resounding testament to the power of scientific validation, delivering an array of life-enhancing benefits that resonate far and wide.

Other benefits

Pilates is a form of exercise that offers numerous benefits for both men and women. While it is often associated with women, it is important to note that Pilates can be highly beneficial for men as well. Stated below are some of the benefits of Pilates for men:

Improved Core Strength: Pilates places a strong emphasis on strengthening the core muscles, including the abdominal muscles, oblique, and lower back. This can lead to better posture, stability, and overall core strength, which is important for everyday activities and athletic performance.

Enhanced Flexibility: Pilates incorporates a range of stretching exercises that can help improve flexibility in the muscles and joints. This increased flexibility can reduce the risk of injury and improve overall mobility.

Increased Body Awareness: Pilates encourages mindfulness and body awareness. Men who practice Pilates often become more in tune with their bodies, which can lead to better movement patterns, posture, and balance.

Improved Posture: Many men suffer from poor posture due to factors such as long hours of sitting at a desk. Pilates can help correct postural imbalances and promote a more upright and natural posture.

Better Balance and Coordination: Pilates exercises often involve precise movements that require coordination and balance. This can help men improve their overall balance and coordination, which can be particularly beneficial for sports and activities that require agility.

Injury Prevention: Pilates focuses on strengthening the muscles around joints, which can help prevent injuries, especially in areas like the knees, hips, and shoulders. It can also aid in the recovery process for those who have experienced injuries.

Stress Reduction: Pilates incorporates deep breathing and relaxation techniques, which can help reduce stress and promote a sense of calm and well-being.

Increased Muscle Tone: While Pilates is not primarily a muscle-building workout, it can help improve muscle tone and definition, especially in the core, legs, and arms.

Enhanced Athletic Performance: Many athletes, including professional athletes, incorporate Pilates into their training routines to improve their strength, flexibility, and overall performance in their respective sports.

Rehabilitation: Pilates can be an effective part of physical therapy and rehabilitation programs. It can help individuals recover from injuries and surgeries by providing gentle yet effective exercise options.

Better Spinal Health: Pilates exercises can help alleviate back pain and improve spinal health by strengthening the muscles that support the spine and promoting better alignment.

Increased Energy Levels: Regular Pilates practice can boost energy levels and leave individuals feeling invigorated.

Printed in Great Britain
by Amazon